Ridiculously Simplified Rheumatology!

Vol 2: The Bone A Fide story of Mr. Osteo and Mrs. Porosis

Dr. Jaya Sonkar, MD, MPH

HOBBIES AND HAPPINESS CREATIONS
Texas, USA

Published by Hobbies and Happiness Creations 2024

ISBN: 978-1-967694-44-0
LCCN: 2026901363

DEDICATION

This book is dedicated to
my daughter
Ms. Riya Agarwal

PREFACE

Bones tell stories.
They whisper tales of our journeys, our nutrition, our hormones, our joys, and our falls. Yet, for most people, bone health remains an invisible topic—until a fracture makes it suddenly real.

I wrote "Mr. Osteo and Mrs. Porosis: A Bone-A-Fide Love Story" to change that. This little book is my attempt to bring medical science out of the clinic and into everyday life, through a lighthearted story that makes you smile *and* think.

In my years as a rheumatologist and geriatrician, I have met countless "Mr. Osteos" and "Mrs. Porosises." They are the people behind every scan, every fracture, every cautious step. Their stories remind me that bone health isn't just about calcium and medications, it's about awareness, prevention, and dignity in aging.

If this story makes you pause before skipping your supplements, if it nudges you to take a walk in the sun, or even if it simply makes you laugh while learning, then it has done its job.

Here's to stronger bones, brighter spirits, and no more dancing on slippery floors!

DISCLAIMER

This story is written in a simple, humorous way to help readers understand osteoporosis and bone health.

It is not intended for medical diagnosis or scientific reference. Always consult your healthcare provider for personalized medical advice.

Written and delightfully simplified for public health education by Dr. Jaya Sonkar, MD, MPH.

Once Upon a Spine...

In a cozy neighborhood lived a cheerful couple — Mr. Osteo, age 70, and his lively wife Mrs. Porosis, age 65.

They were the kind of couple who finished each other’s sentences — and snacks. Life was smooth... until one day it got a little 'bumpy'.

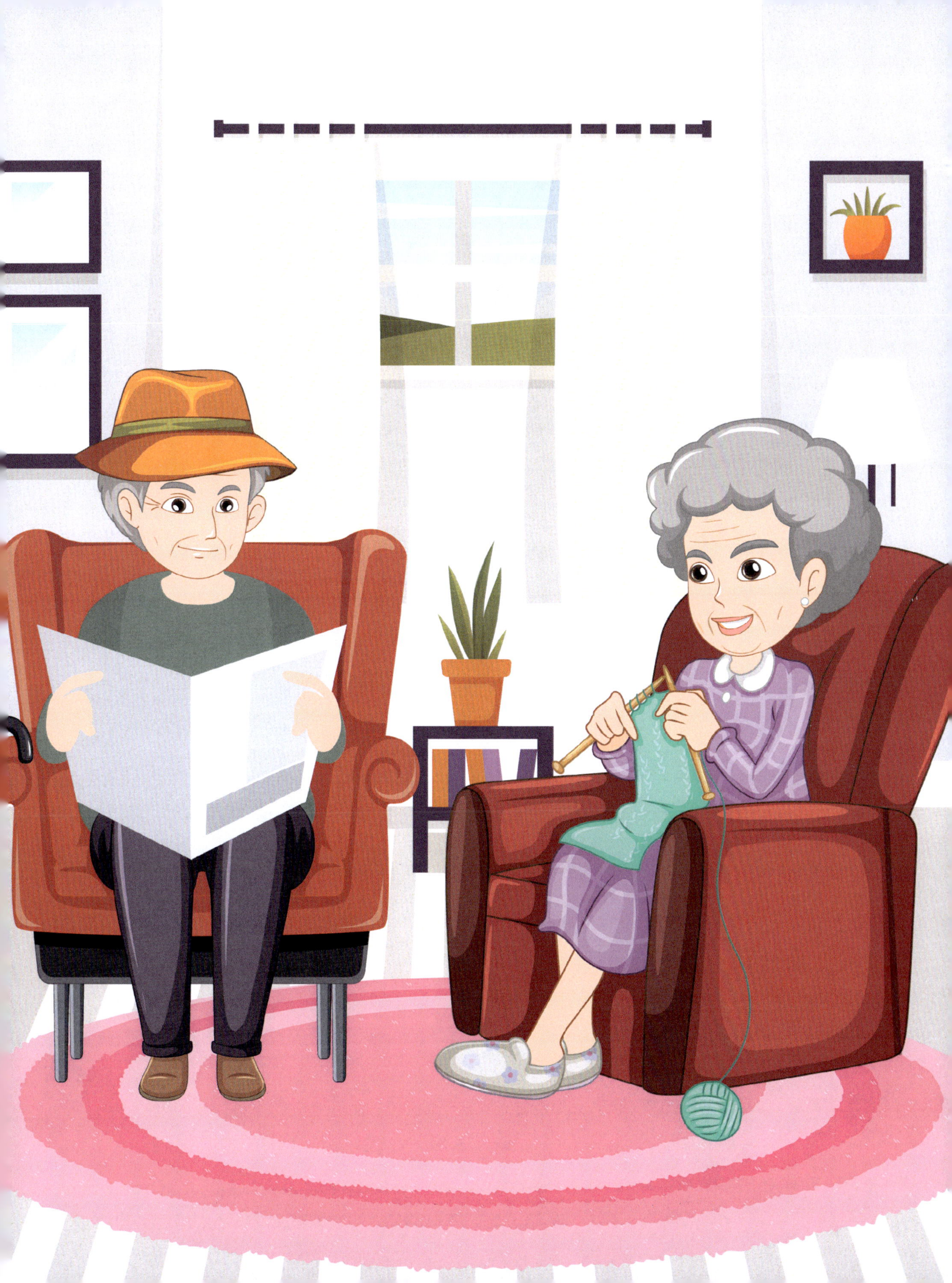

The Road Trip Lesson

Mr. Osteo had to attend a medical conference by the boathouse, a four-hour drive away. On the way, he noticed road work. Huge machines dug small pits but somehow removed giant chunks of road. Then another machine rolled in and made it all smooth again.

He chuckled, “Tiny hole, massive repair — must be the government budget at work.” He didn’t know that the same thing was happening quietly inside our bones every day.

TINY HOLES, BIG REPAIR,
JUST LIKE INSIDE OUR BONES!

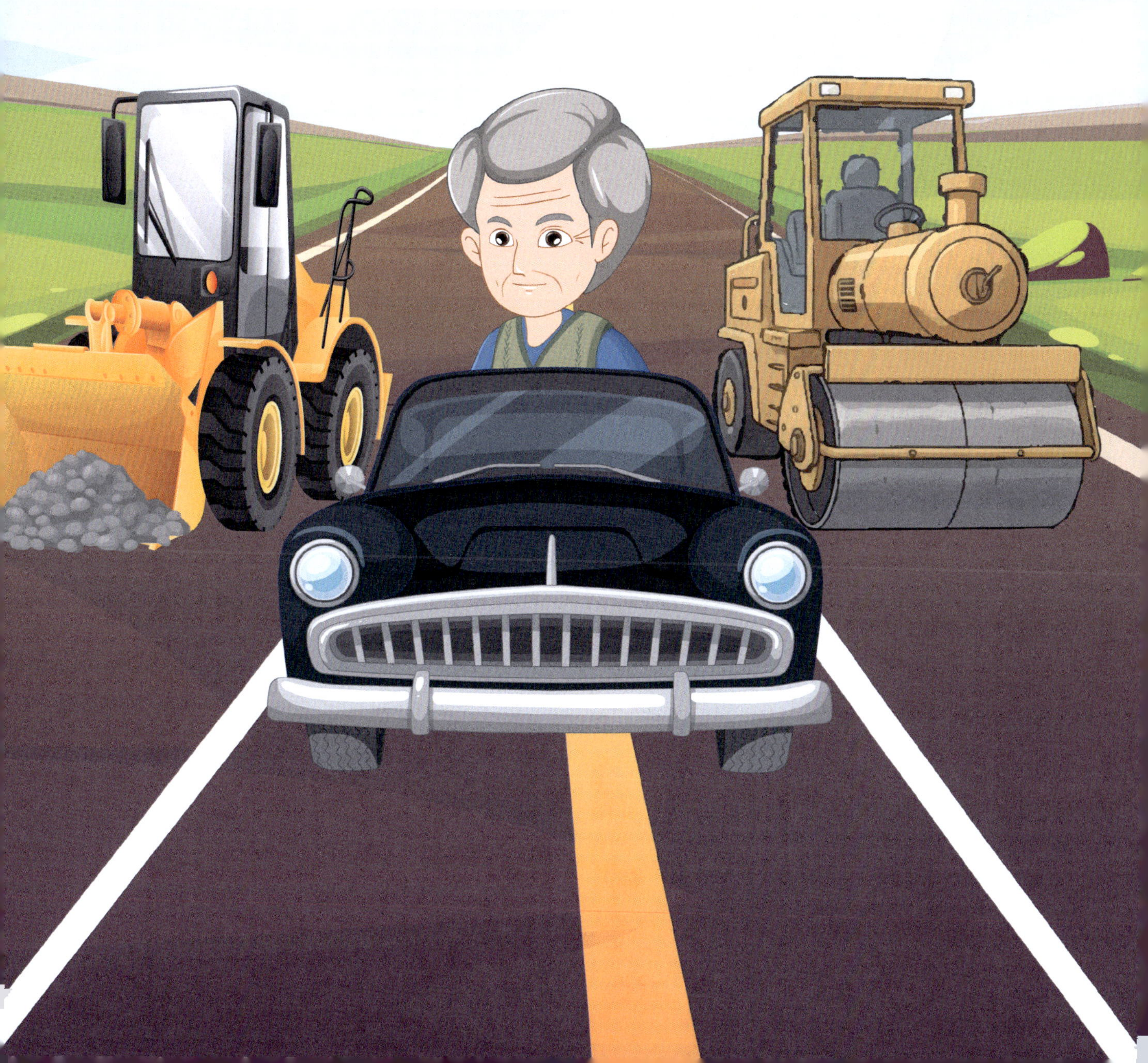

The Slip

When he came home, Mrs. Porosis was cooking her favorite meal, humming an old song, when 'splat!' one sneaky drop of oil betrayed her.

She slipped, fell, and cried out, “Oh, my hip!”

They rushed to the ER.

An X-ray confirmed a **hip fracture**, and surgery followed.

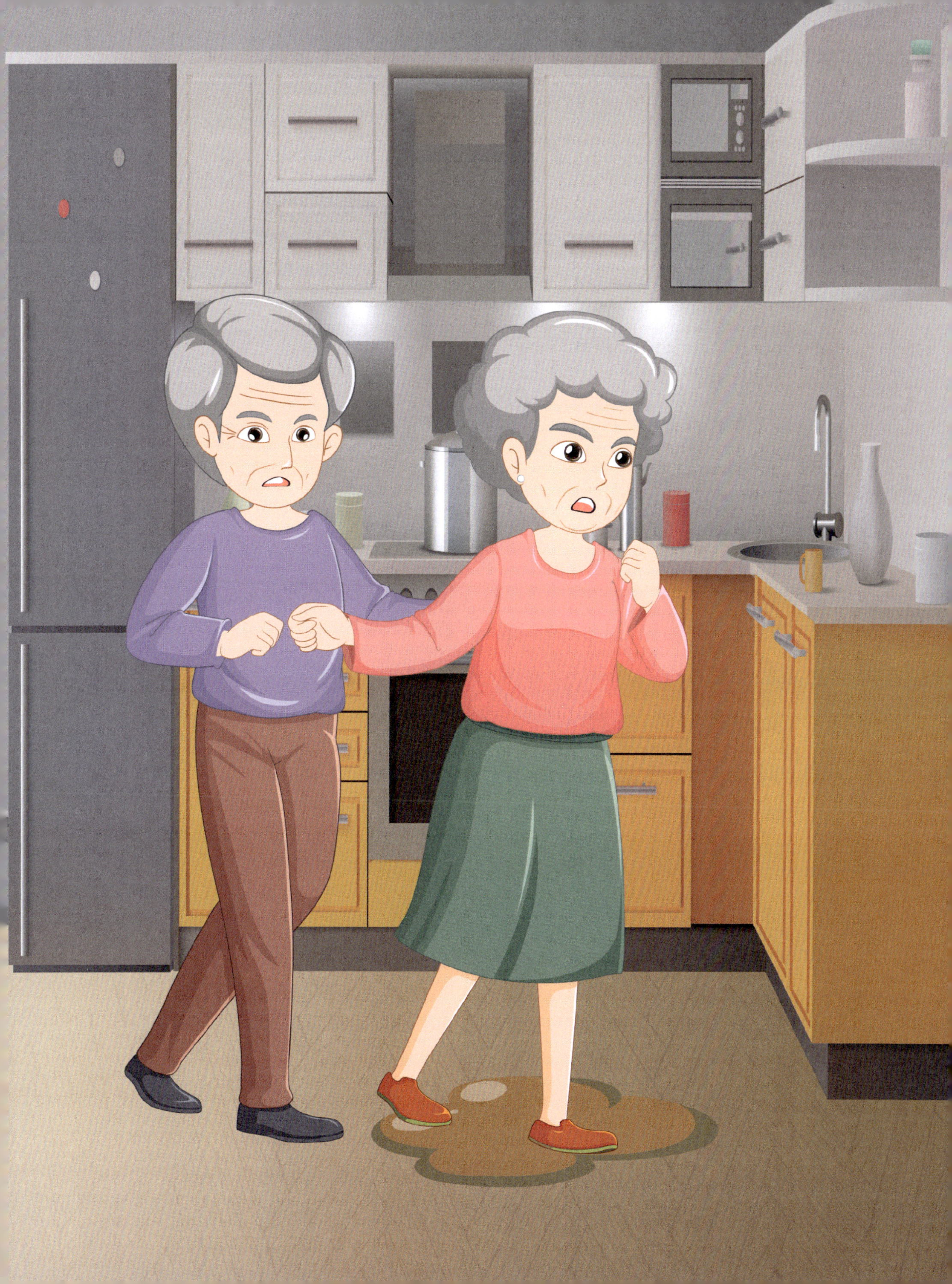

The Diagnosis

After the operation, the doctor ordered a DEXA scan.

“Mrs. Porosis,” he said gently, “your **T-score is below –2.5**. That means **osteoporosis** — your bones have become porous and fragile.”

Mr. Osteo blinked. “Porous bones? Like Swiss cheese?”

The doctor smiled. “Exactly. Except cheese tastes better.”

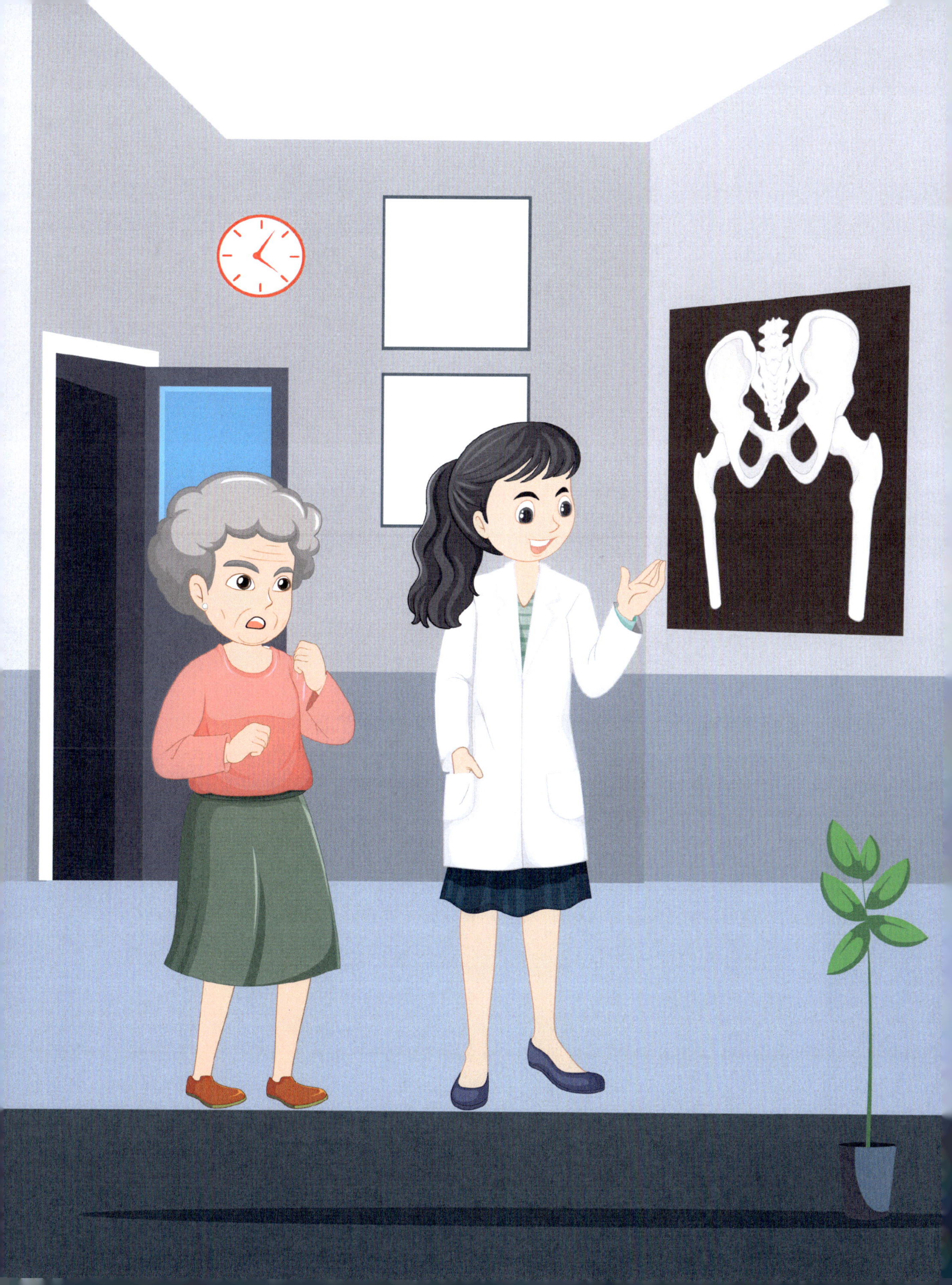

Calcium & Vitamin D — the Dynamic Duo

“Have you been taking calcium and vitamin D?” the doctor asked.

Mrs. Porosis sighed, “Doctor, I’m lactose intolerant. Milk and I aren’t friends.”

“That’s fine,” he said. “We’ll use supplements. Remember:

Vitamin D_2: comes from plants,
Vitamin D_3: from animal sources, and D_3 works a bit better.

Some people take vitamin K_2 with it, but it’s not always needed. Just don’t overdo calcium — too much can be as tricky as too little.”

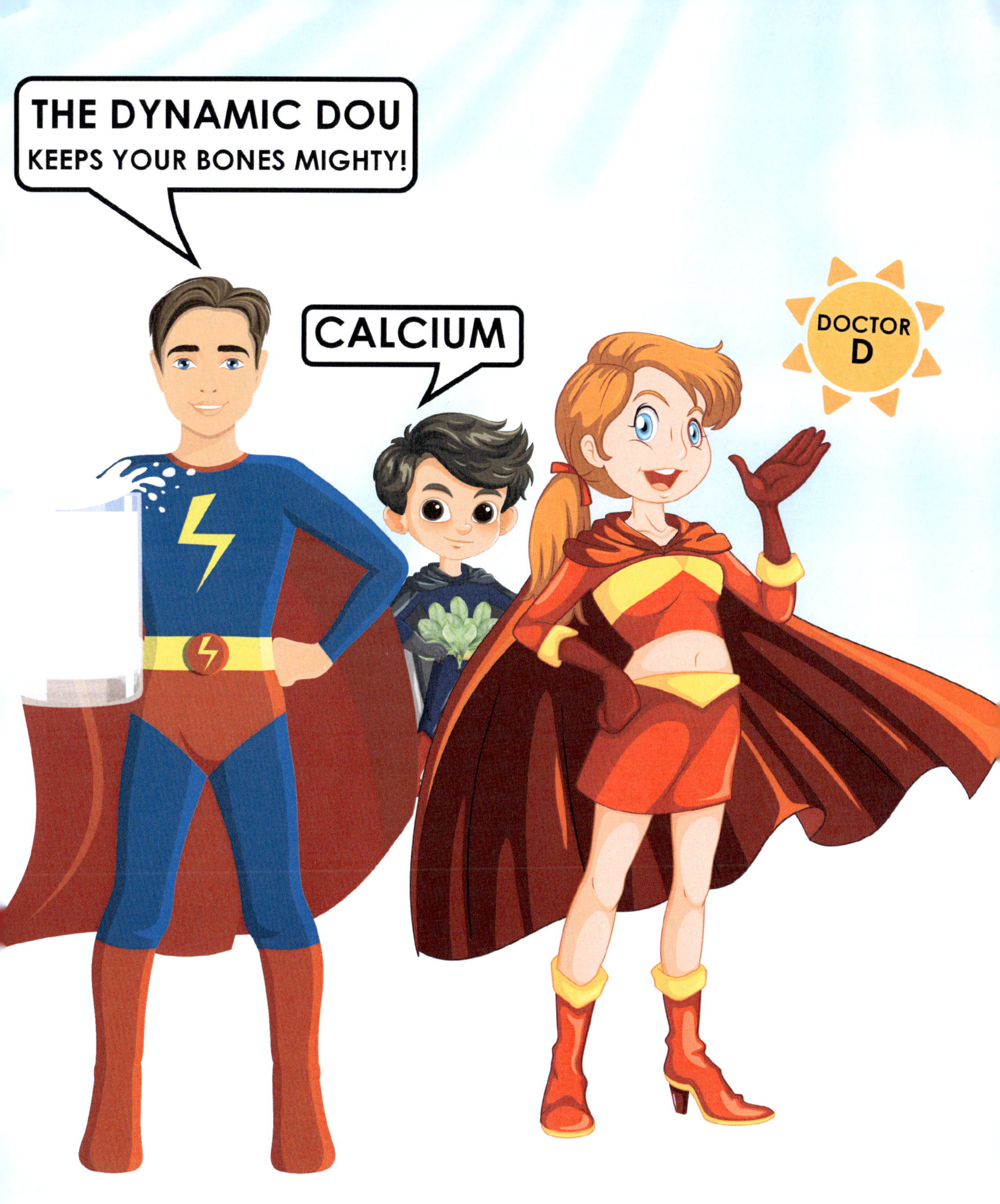
THE DYNAMIC DOU
KEEPS YOUR BONES MIGHTY!
CALCIUM
DOCTOR
D

Bone Road Repair 101

"Think of bones like the road you saw," said the doctor.

"The osteoclasts are like the crew that cuts old pitted road — they break down bone. The osteoblasts are the ones that lay new road — they build bone."

"As we age, the demolition crew works just fine while the builders slow down. And our bones weaken and holes start forming."

MEET YOUR ROAD CREW

REPAIR IN PROGRESS 24/7!

BONE ROAD REPAIR 101

DEMOLATION TEAM

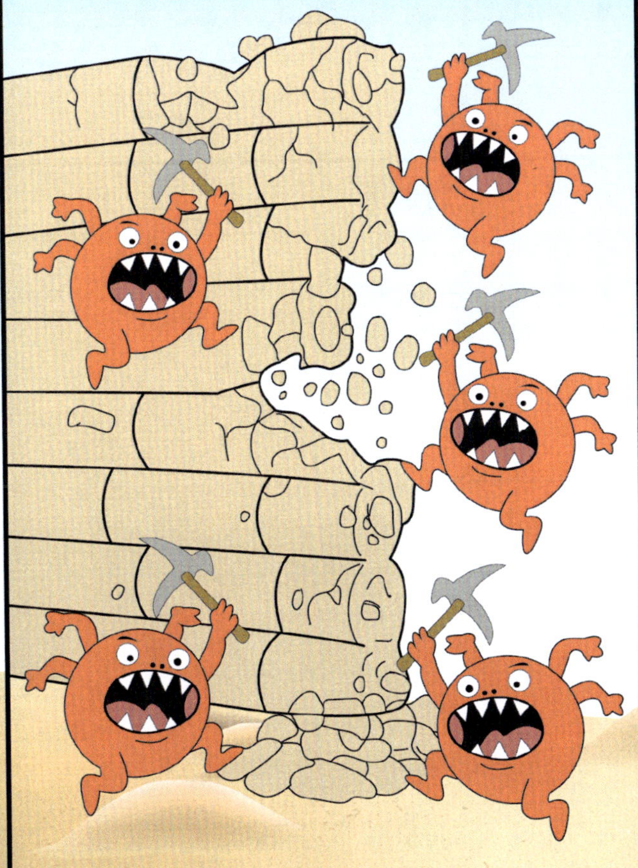

CONSTRUCTION TEAM

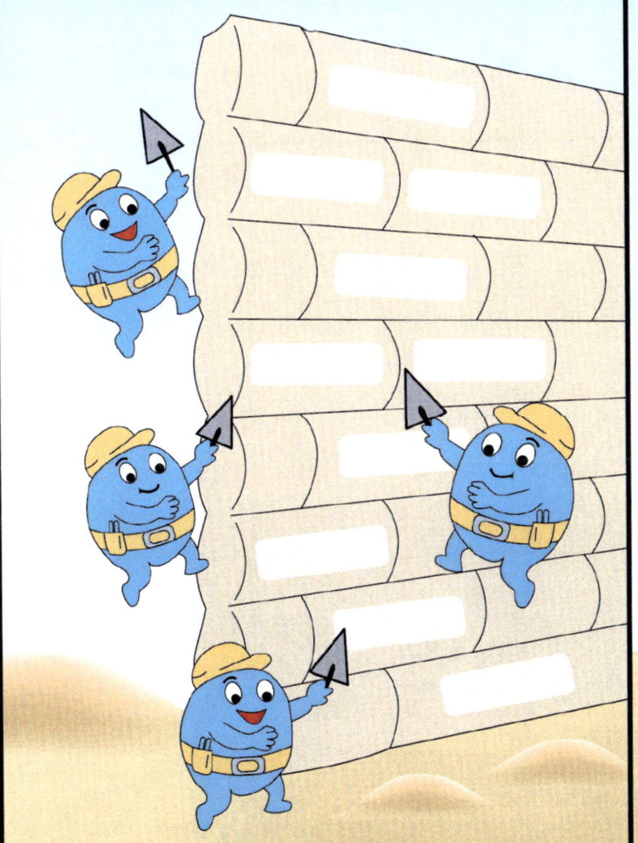

The Culprits Behind the Cracks

The doctor ticked them off one by one:

Aging (can't fight that one!)
Low calcium or vitamin D
Family history of osteoporosis or fractures
Rheumatoid arthritis
Smoking or alcohol
Steroids(they speed up bone loss)
Diabetes or hormone disorders

Mr. Osteo nodded, "Ah, her mother broke her hip too!"

The doctor smiled, "Exactly, sometimes bones follow family traditions."

Mrs. Porosis rolled her eyes. "Great, genetics gave me curly hair *and* weak bones."

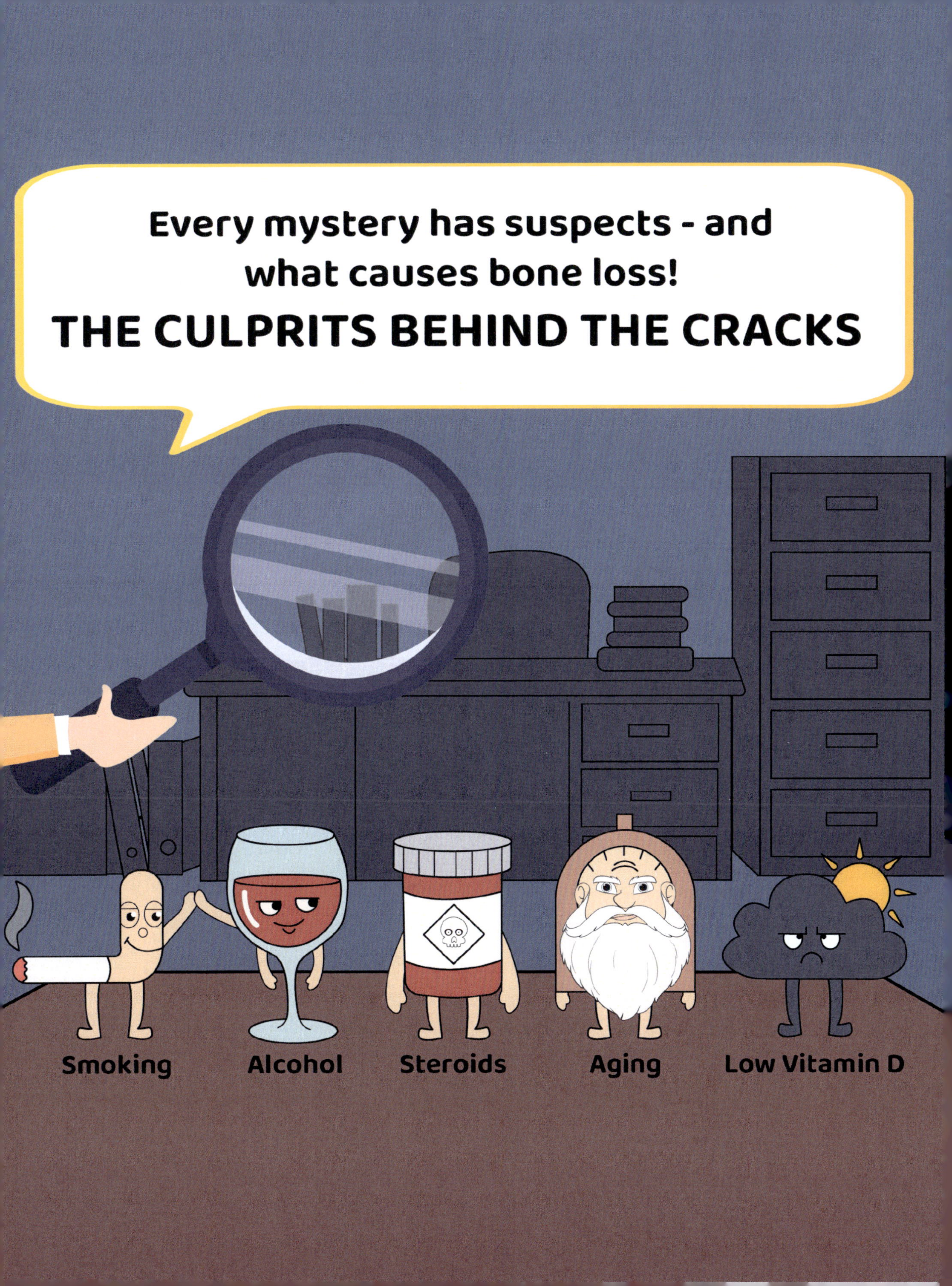
Every mystery has suspects - and what causes bone loss!
THE CULPRITS BEHIND THE CRACKS
Smoking
Alcohol
Steroids
Aging
Low Vitamin D

Meet Osteopenia — the Warning Sister

“Before osteoporosis,” the doctor explained, “comes osteopenia, the little sister who politely warns you, “Hey, start working on those bones!”

Here’s how to keep her happy:

- Weight-bearing exercise (walk, dance, climb stairs)
- Resistance training (light weights, bands)
- Sunlight for vitamin D
- Calcium + vitamin D regularly
- No smoking, and go easy on the wine

Mrs. Porosis grinned, “So the prescription is dancing, sunshine, and groceries? I can do that!”

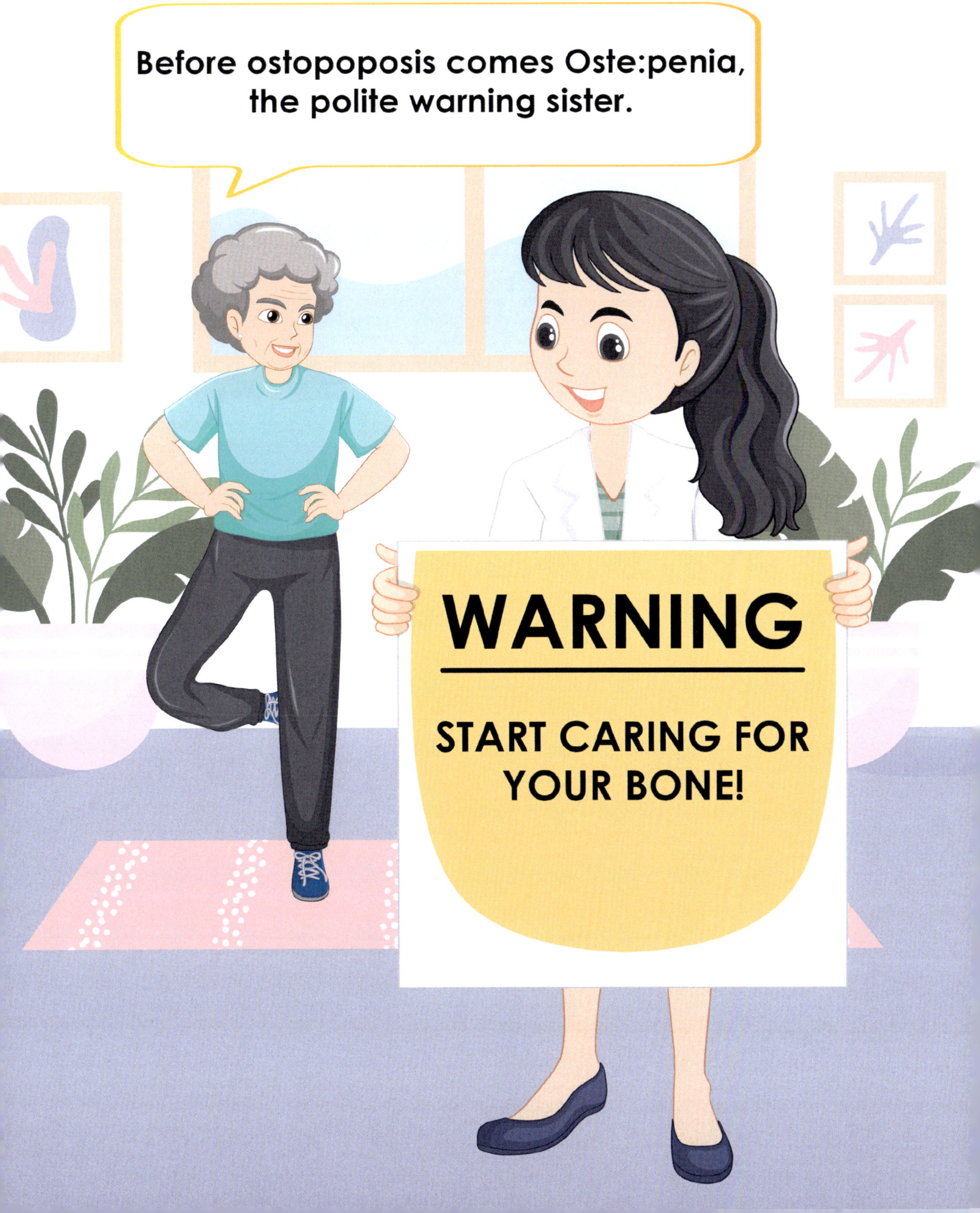
Before ostopoposis comes Oste:penia,
the polite warning sister.
WARNING
START CARING FOR
YOUR BONE!

The Bone Squad

1. Bisphosphonates: Tell the bone-cutters to slow down. Fewer holes, stronger road. Rarely, they may cause jaw or unusual fractures with long use, but overall they're dependable.

2. Denosumab (Prolia): Blocks the troublemaker **RANK ligand**, which usually traps our bone-protector **osteoprotegerin**.

Once RANK ligand is stopped, osteoprotegerin can freely protect bones and let builders rebuild.

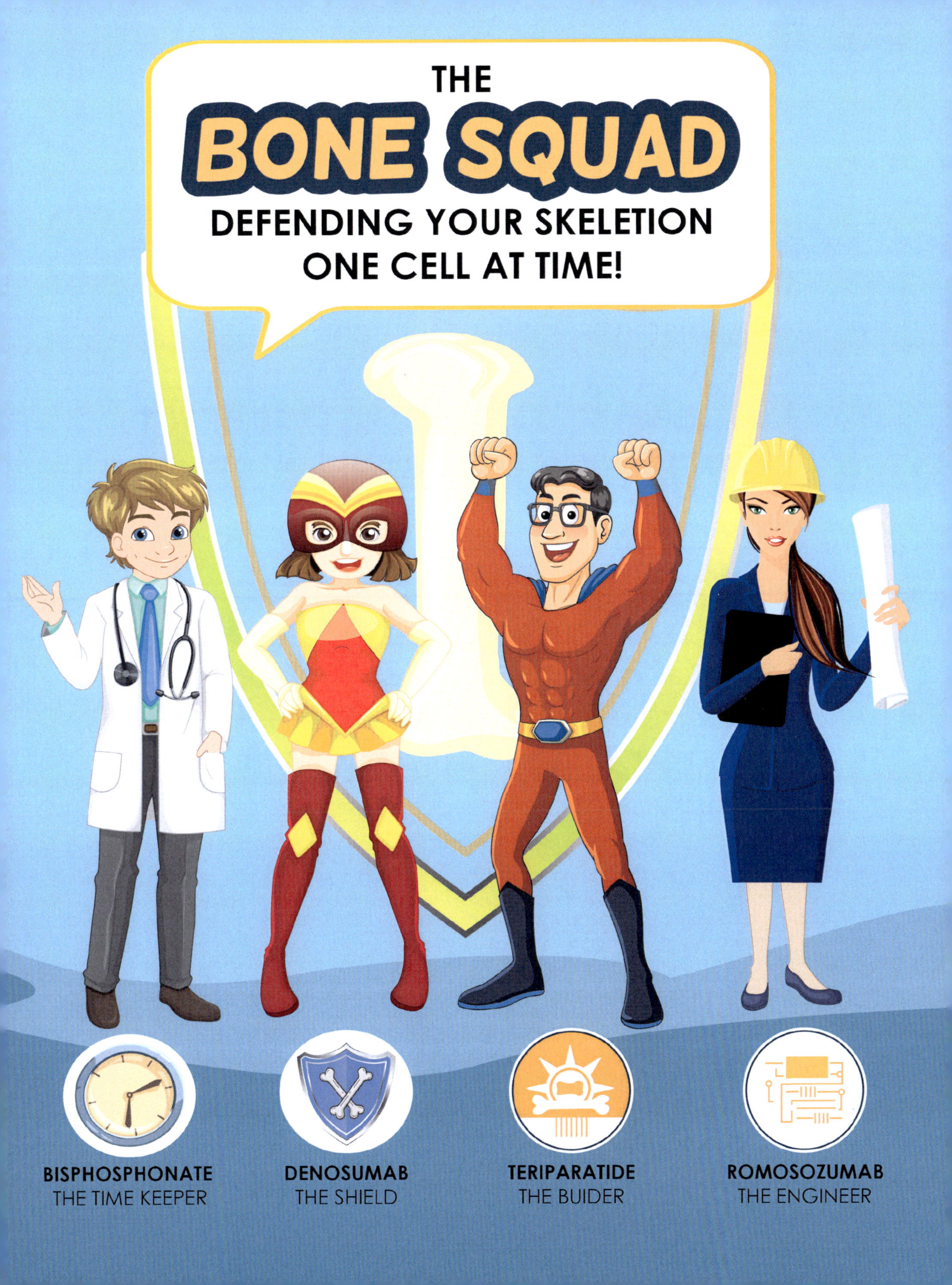
THE
BONE SQUAD
DEFENDING YOUR SKELETION
ONE CELL AT TIME!
BISPHOSPHONATE
THE TIME KEEPER
DENOSUMAB
THE SHIELD
TERIPARATIDE
THE BUIDER
ROMOSOZUMAB
THE ENGINEER

3. Teriparatide & Abaloparatide: The “bone-builder boosters.” They energize osteoblasts to make new bone.

Not used for teenagers, people with growing bones, high calcium, or certain cancers.

4. Romosozumab: Blocks "sclerostin", allowing faster bone formation. But it can increase risk of clots, stroke, or heart attack, so avoid if you’ve had these in the past year. Always discuss with your doctor.

Raloxifene (SERM) may also help in certain situation

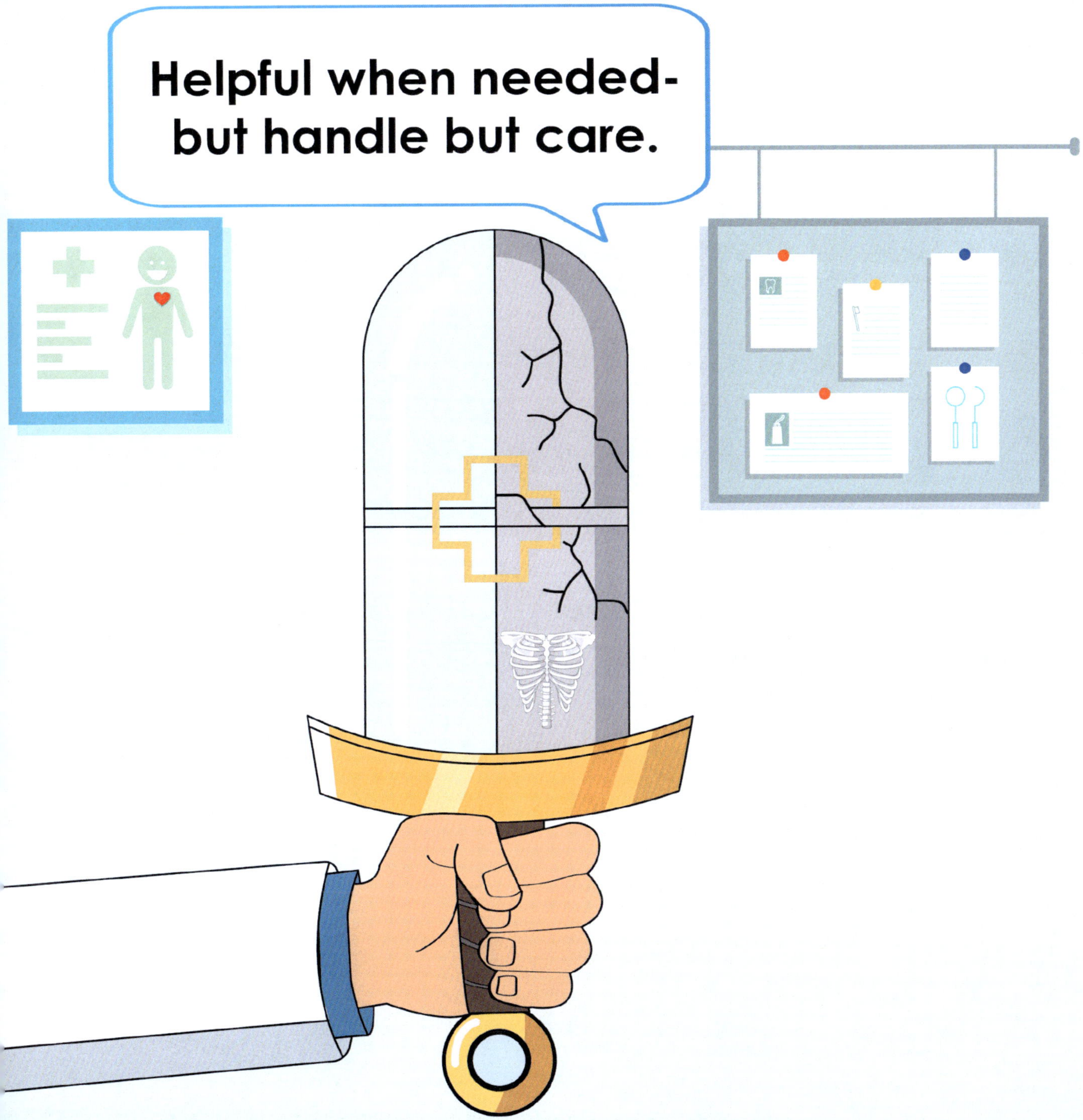

STEROIDS: THE DOUBLE-EDGED SWORD

A Word About Steroids

“Steroids,” said the doctor seriously, “can quietly steal calcium from your bones if taken for long periods. Even small daily doses can increase osteoporosis risk.”

Mrs. Porosis gasped, “So those tiny pills pack a punch!”

“Exactly,” he said, “they’re double-edged swords — helpful when needed, but we use them
wisely.”

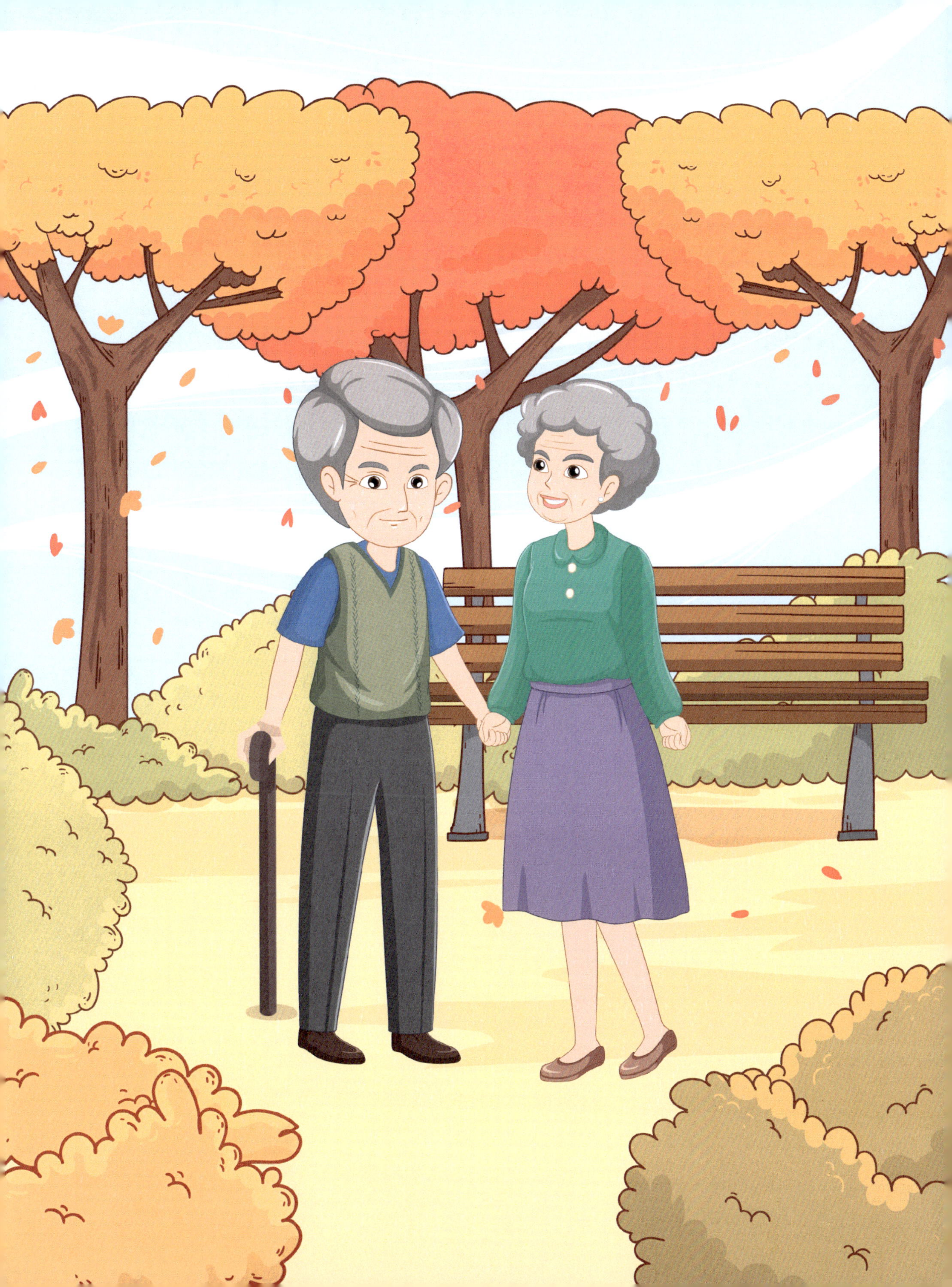

Strong Bones, Strong Life

As they headed home, the doctor smiled, "Bones are like roads, they need maintenance, nutrients, and care. Keep them strong with exercise, calcium, vitamin D, and healthy habits."

Mr. Osteo nodded, "No potholes in love, no potholes in bones."

Mrs. Porosis laughed, "And no dancing on slippery floors!"

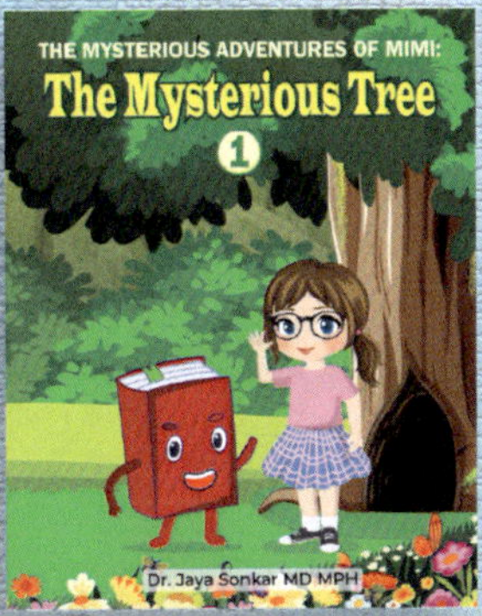
THE MYSTERIOUS ADVENTURES OF MIMI:
The Mysterious Tree
1
Dr. Jaya Sonkar MD MPH

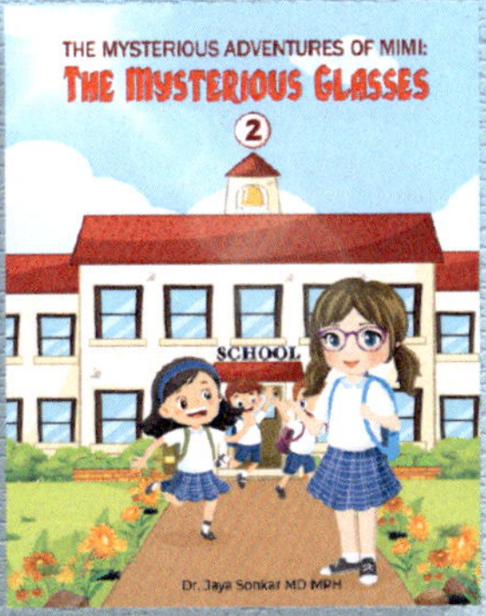
THE MYSTERIOUS ADVENTURES OF MIMI:
THE MYSTERIOUS GLASSES
2
SCHOOL
Dr. Jaya Sonkar MD MPH

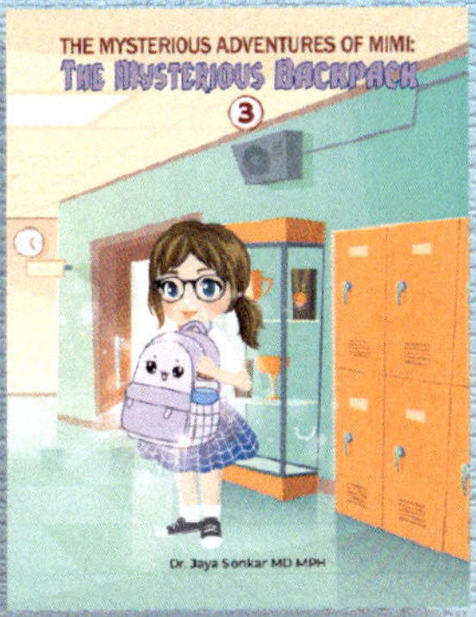
THE MYSTERIOUS ADVENTURES OF MIMI:
THE MYSTERIOUS BACKPACK
3
Dr. Jaya Sonkar MD MPH

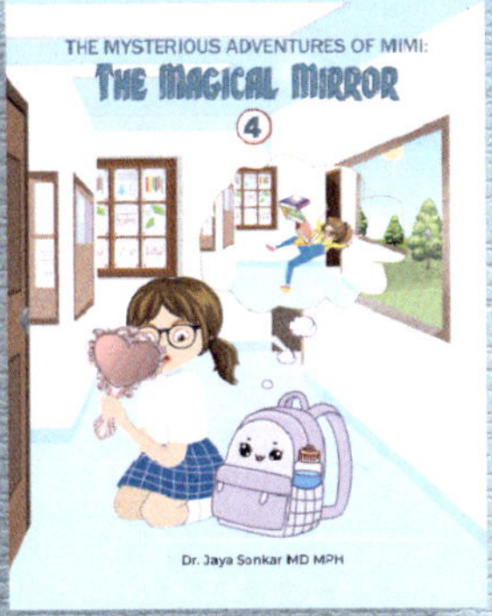
THE MYSTERIOUS ADVENTURES OF MIMI:
THE MAGICAL MIRROR
4
Dr. Jaya Sonkar MD MPH

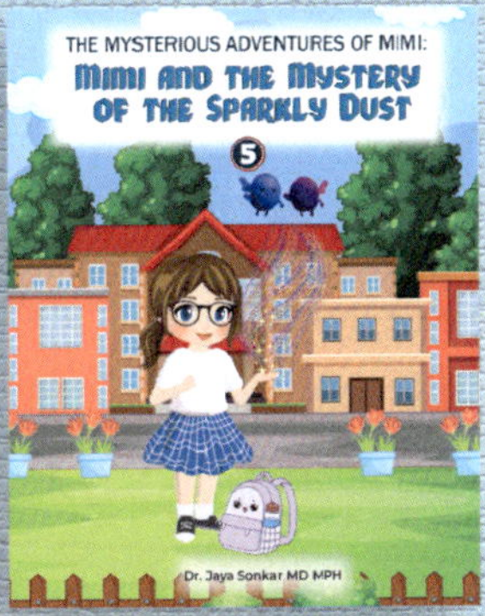
THE MYSTERIOUS ADVENTURES OF MIMI:
MIMI AND THE MYSTERY OF THE SPARKLY DUST
5
Dr. Jaya Sonkar MD MPH

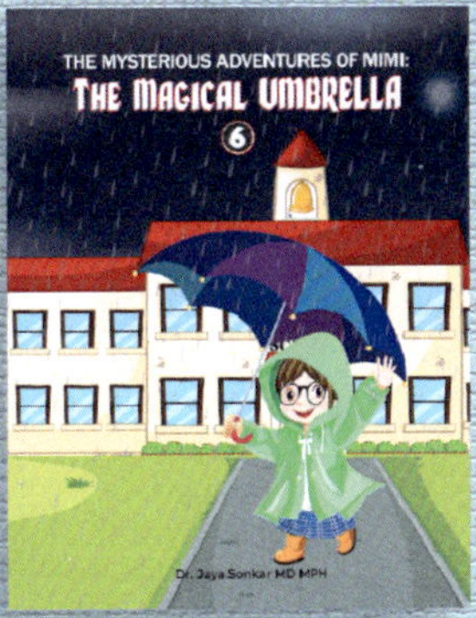
THE MYSTERIOUS ADVENTURES OF MIMI:
THE MAGICAL UMBRELLA
6
Dr. Jaya Sonkar MD MPH

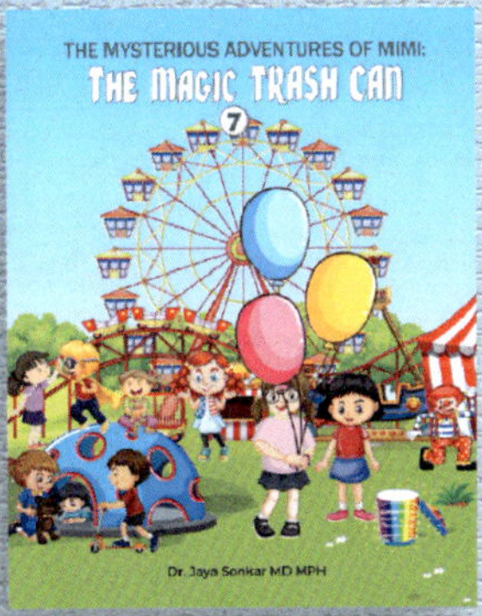
THE MYSTERIOUS ADVENTURES OF MIMI:
THE MAGIC TRASH CAN
7
Dr. Jaya Sonkar MD MPH

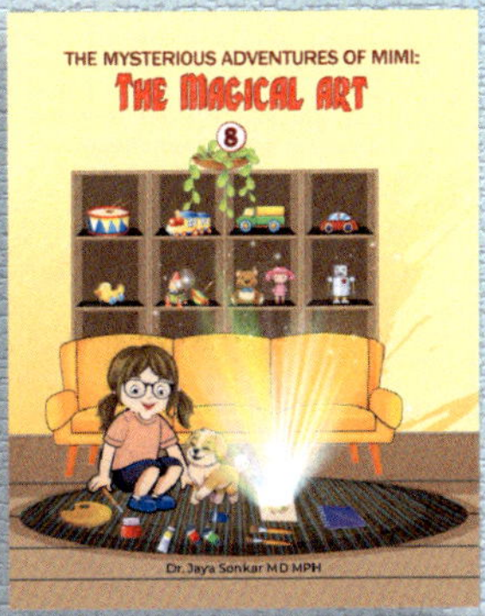
THE MYSTERIOUS ADVENTURES OF MIMI:
THE MAGICAL ART
8
Dr. Jaya Sonkar MD MPH

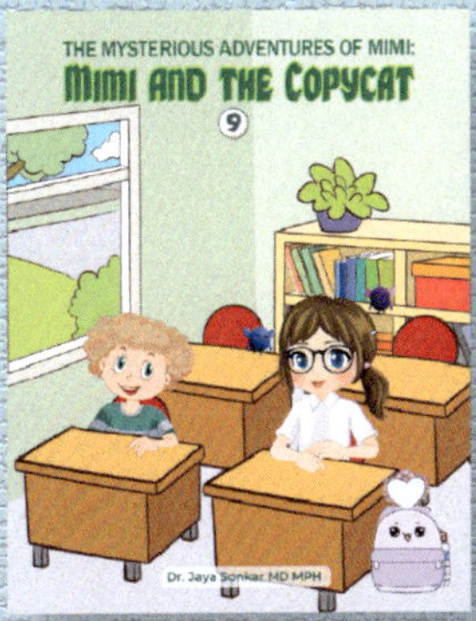
THE MYSTERIOUS ADVENTURES OF MIMI:
MIMI AND THE COPYCAT
9
Dr. Jaya Sonkar MD MPH

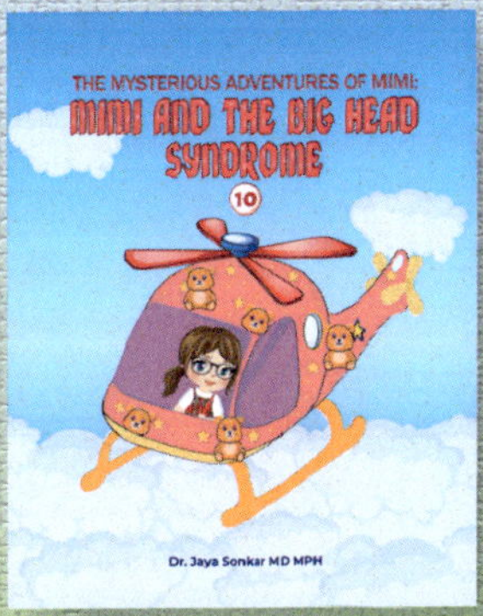
THE MYSTERIOUS ADVENTURES OF MIMI:
MIMI AND THE BIG HEAD SYNDROME
10
Dr. Jaya Sonkar MD MPH

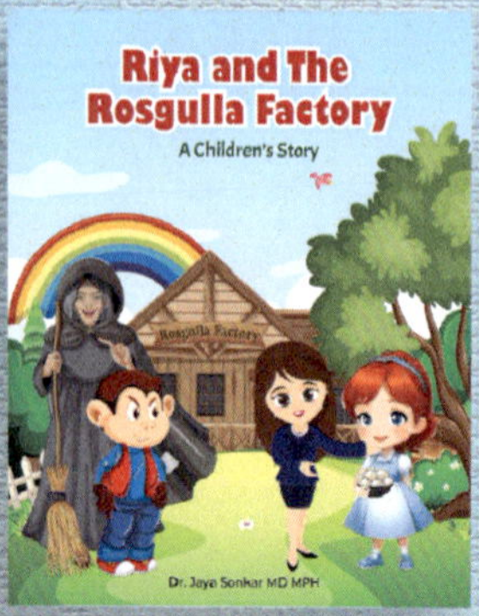
Riya and The Rosgulla Factory
A Children's Story
Rosgulla Factory
Dr. Jaya Sonkar MD MPH

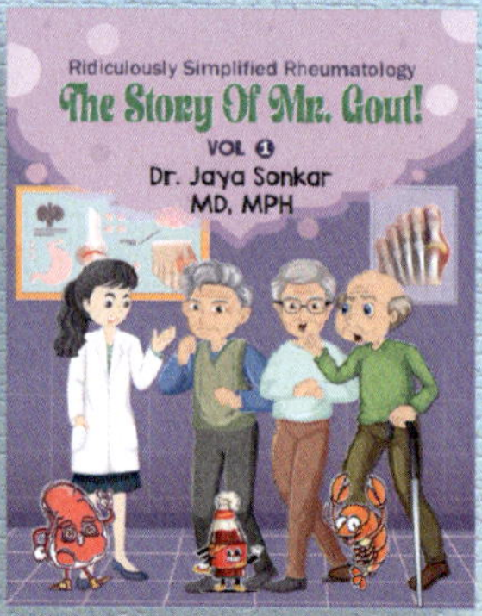
Ridiculously Simplified Rheumatology
The Story Of Mr. Gout!
VOL 1
Dr. Jaya Sonkar
MD, MPH

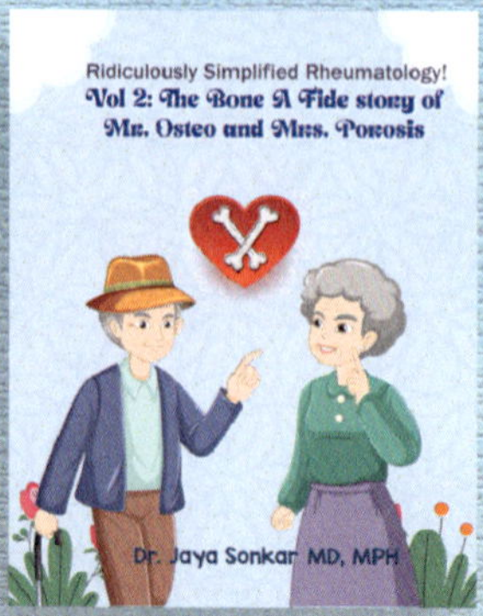
Ridiculously Simplified Rheumatology!
Vol 2: The Bone A Fide story of
Mr. Osteo and Mrs. Porosis
Dr. Jaya Sonkar MD, MPH

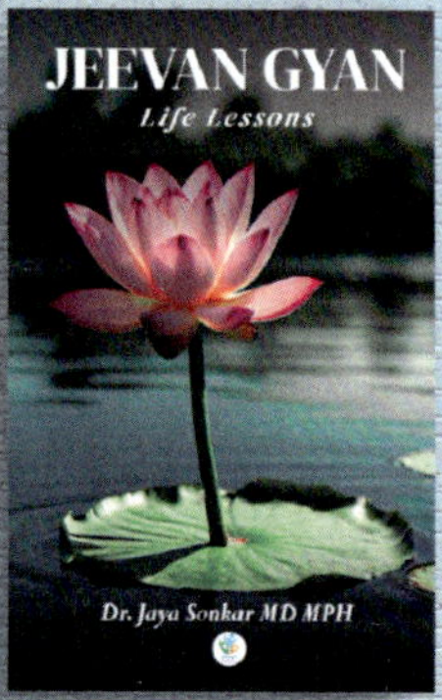
JEEVAN GYAN
Life Lessons
Dr. Jaya Sonkar MD MPH

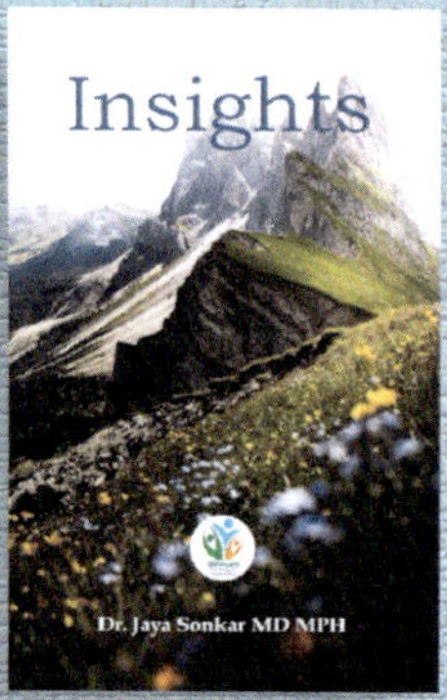
Insights
Dr. Jaya Sonkar MD MPH

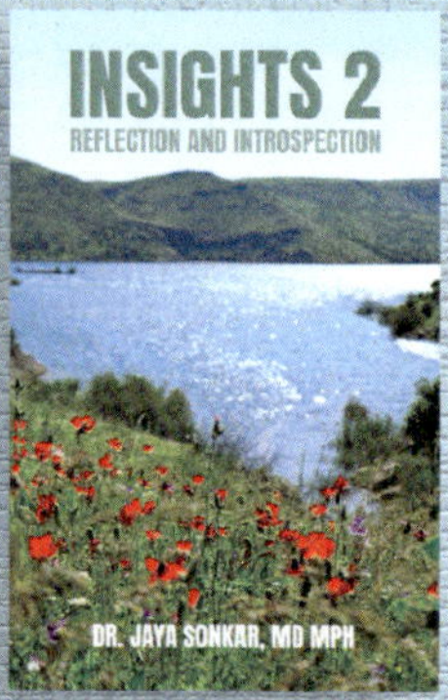
INSIGHTS 2
REFLECTION AND INTROSPECTION
DR. JAYA SONKAR, MD MPH

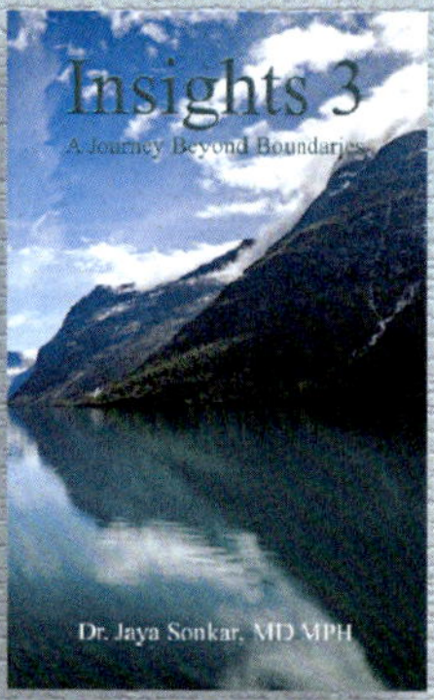
Insights 3
A Journey Beyond Boundaries
Dr. Jaya Sonkar, MD MPH

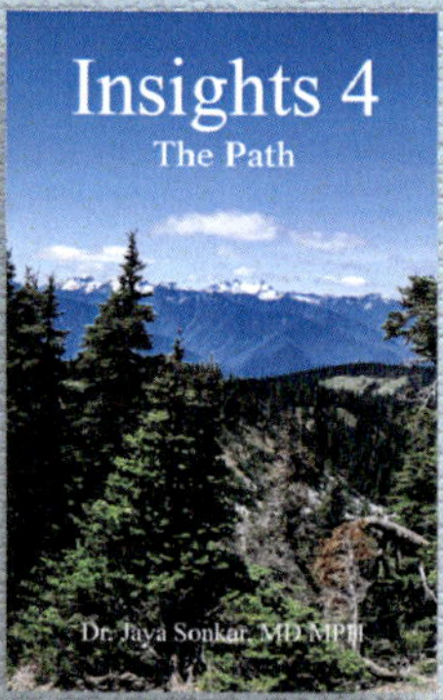
Insights 4
The Path
Dr. Jaya Sonkar, MD MPH

Made in United States
Orlando, FL
05 November 2026

90230157R00019